MW01281773

WHOLE DIET 30 DAYS

─ ─ ─ ─ ─ ❧ ❧ ❧ ❧ ─ ─ ─ ─ ─

Find out your vitality with this ultimate clean-eating program for 30 days and unleash your energy

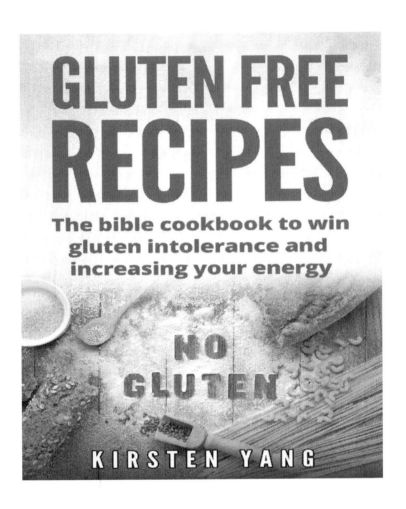

Do you have celiac disease or gluten sensitivity?

This book will show you just how tasty a gluten- free diet can be

GET YOUR COPY NOW

https://goo.gl/kf1fJo

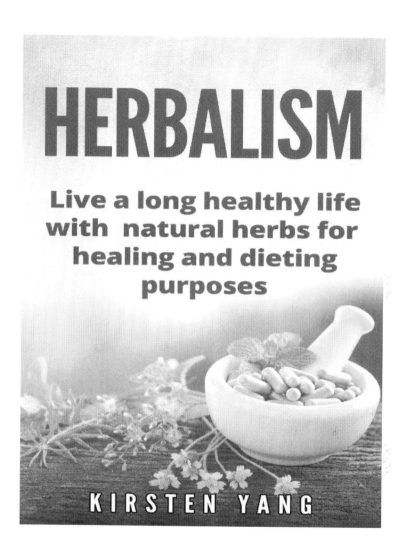

HERBALISM

Live a long healthy life with natural herbs for healing and dieting purposes

KIRSTEN YANG

Discover the enormous potential of herbs for healing and dieting purposes

GET YOUR COPY NOW

https://goo.gl/7KNNHA

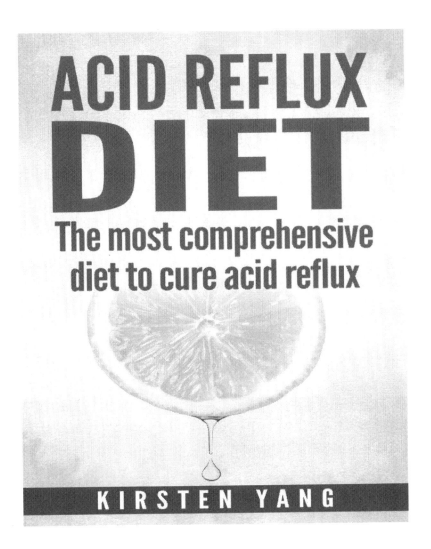

Do you wanna stop the acid reflux with the ultimate cookbook and feel free to talk with people!?

GET YOUR COPY NOW

https://goo.gl/GFyrH1

ZERO SUGAR
DIET
Burn belly fat instantly and get a killer body

KIRSTEN YANG

Do You Want To Get a Killer Body Instantly?!

GET YOUR COPY NOW

https://goo.gl/UbChfX

© Copyright 2017 by Kirsten Yang - All rights reserved.

The follow eBook is reproduced below with the goal of providing information that is as accurate and reliable as possible. Regardless, purchasing this eBook can be seen as consent to the fact that both the publisher and the author of this book are in no way experts on the topics discussed within and that any recommendations or suggestions that are made herein are for entertainment purposes only.

Professionals should be consulted as needed prior to undertaking any of the action endorsed herein.

This declaration is deemed fair and valid by both the American Bar Association and the Committee of Publishers Association and is legally binding throughout the United States.

If you would like to share this book with another person, please purchase an additional copy for each recipient. Thank you for respecting the hard work of this author. Otherwise, the transmission, duplication or reproduction of any of the following work including specific information will be considered an illegal act irrespective of if it is done electronically or in print. This extends to creating a secondary or tertiary copy of the work or a recorded copy and is only allowed with express written consent from the Publisher. All additional right reserved.

The information in the following pages is broadly considered to be a truthful and accurate account of facts and as such any inattention, use or misuse of the information in question by the reader will render any resulting actions solely under their purview. There are no scenarios in which the publisher or the original author of this work can be in any fashion deemed liable for any hardship or damages that may befall them after undertaking information described herein.

Additionally, the information in the following pages is intended only for informational purposes and should thus be thought of as universal. As befitting its nature, it is presented without assurance regarding its prolonged validity or interim quality. Trademarks that are mentioned are done without written consent and can in no way be considered an endorsement from the trademark holder.

Table of Contents

Introduction

— — — — — ✍ ✍ ✍ ✍ — — — — —

If asked, a good percentage of people would agree that their eating habits could use a healthy upgrade.

The modern diet consists of quick and easy processed foods that are often fattening and packed with unhealthy carbohydrates. In our fast-paced society, people often prepare foods that are convenient and easy to make to fit into their busy schedules.

In order to make true, lasting changes in their eating habits, people need to search for the best diet plans. The word "best" refers to diet plans that give dieters the tools and resources they need to switch from unhealthy foods to whole food choices over time. Some people have to make sudden dietary changes in the case of serious health conditions, such as heart disease, celiac disease, and diabetes.

Most people, however, can start ridding themselves of excess food baggage on their shelves and begin replacing them with sprouted grains, fresh produce, and healthy fat.

Diets that are rich in whole foods are the best way of eating for good nutritional and physical health. The American Dietary Association's recommendation to switch from refined products to whole grains is a part of the national effort to change unhealthy eating habits.

People that focus on eating good carbohydrates, such as fresh produce, whole grains, and eating lean meats, will see a slow and steady improvement in their health and well-being. There is a direct correlation between healthy eating and good heart health, among other health conditions. A whole diet approach to eating often deters people because they believe they do not have the time to prepare healthy foods from scratch.

In addition, people, especially lower-income families, may not be able to afford to buy a lot of expensive produce from the market. Many communities have produced stands or discount stores that provide fresh produce at discounted prices. In addition, many discount food stores offer to produce at prices that are lower than at the more popular food chains.

There are many successful diet plans on the market that already incorporate a whole diet in their principles. A diet plan that involves eating fruit, vegetables, olive oil, beans, whole grains, and fish for a whole diet look promising. This kind of diet is encouraged by health professionals and is shown to be a preventive dietary pattern that reduces the chance of developing serious health conditions.

This effective dietary plan has also been said to promote a healthy metabolism and have great weight loss results. It is easier to make dietary changes when there are a lot of healthy foods from which dieters can choose.

The Whole Diet for 30 days way of eating is a diet plan that implements the principles of eating good whole foods, including organic and free-range meats. The results of this program are undeniable in achieving weight loss and lowering the risk of chronic conditions or serious disease.

Finding the best diet plans on the market are not hard to find or difficult to follow, as many are geared to lifestyle changes. Studies have shown that this kind of incremental approach to dieting helps people to lose weight and maintain it. Diet changes do take a good deal of time and investment, but they can lead to a better q uality of life now and for years to come.

Chapter 1

─ ─ ─ ─ ─ ❧❦❧❦ ─ ─ ─ ─ ─

How to Diet Successfully for 30 Days

Have you ever wondered how to diet successfully? There are several diet plans out there that have been built on a misconception and fabrication, and only a few of them really work.

With that in mind, here are free notes on how to diet successfully. These tips are really simple, but these are also what nutritionists advise everyone that wants to lose weight. Diet is more important than an intense workout in the gym when it comes to losing weight; the best way to lose weight is still to control the food that we are consuming every day.

1.   TO EAT OR NOT TO EAT CARBS

The first tip on how to diet successfully is involved carbohydrates. There are many diet plans that restrict the intake of carbohydrates, but several nutritionists believe that the low intake of carbohydrates does not lead to weight loss.

In actuality, it is the fatty ingredients that we add to the carbohydrates, such as the butter or margarine that we put on our bread and the cheese we put on our pasta, which cause the weight gain.

The good carbohydrates, however, such as bread, breakfast cereals, pasta, and rice actually help give us the daily energy we need while giving us lower calories than alcohol and fat. So in order to lose weight, we need to cut down on the added fats and not the carbs.

2.   STOCK UP ON FRUITS AND VEGETABLES

Fruits and vegetables contain sugars and while we might be skeptical about adding sugar into our diet, fruits and vegetables actually contain the best and natural kind of sugar that they contain fiber, nutrition, and water.

As an added benefit, not only are fruits and vegetables recommended by nutritionists when asked how to diet successfully to lose weight, they also help reduce blood cholesterol and also contain micronutrients that help protect us against diseases such as blood cancer.

3.   NO TO PROCESSED SUGAR

The type of sugar that we should be avoiding, on the other hand, is refined sugar. If there is one thing that will sabotage your whole diet plan, it is refined sugar. Unlike those found in fresh fruits and vegetables, processed sugar contains many fewer nutrients and fiber and adds weight to the body quickly. It is also important to keep drinking water.

There is no limit as to how much water we take daily as it is also q uickly excreted from the body. Not only does water cleanse our bodies, it also, somehow, acts as a replacement for food, and suppresses our hunger pains q uickly. So when you are wondering how to diet successfully, you just simply need to eat a lot of natural, healthy food and drink plenty of water.

Chapter 2

─ ─ ─ ─ ─ ❧❦❧ ─ ─ ─ ─ ─

Making a Day by Day Diet Plan that You can Stick to for 30 Days

Being overweight can cause a lot of problems to an individual. People who are overweight often feel weak and sluggish. Individuals who have weight problems also suffer from low confidence, and even depression.

Now, by finding an ideal day by day diet and changing what and when you eat, can help you get rid of your excess body fats and give you more self-confidence. By undergoing fat burning diet, you will be able to have enough energy that you can spend for performing your daily activities.

You'll be able to have enough strength; you'll be able to think clearer and much better. And most of all, by going on a day by day diet program, you'll feel better about yourself.

Changing your day by day diet will initially be a pain. Shifting from what you're used to eating to what you should eat is very difficult. Nevertheless, it is also easy to create and/or find an ideal fat burning diet that is easy to follow and one which will fit right into your life.

When you're just beginning to go on a day by day diet plan, make sure to start with a simple menu. Don't try to change your whole diet in one week; if you do this, it will be hard for you to stick to your fat burning diet plan.

Make sure to change your daily diet gradually for the period of at least 30 days, this way, it will be easier for you to adapt to your new eating habit.

Slowly, try to cut down on your intake of foods that are responsible for your excess body fats such as meat, crackers, ice cream, cakes, etc.

Chapter 3

— — — — — ❦❧ — — — —

The Importance of Staying Committed to Your Diet

Dieting is a process which involves a great deal of willpower. This is because a number of restrictions exist during the duration of the plan. This is the reason why many people do not succeed when it is concerned with their diet plans.

This has made many people dread the idea of dieting as they always have the dumb intuition that they would not be able to follow the routine resulting in many diet plans to fail even before they are started. Many people fail to understand that healthy dieting does not refer to starving.

This is one major reason for many people to not take up dieting as they think they will have to completely stay away from food which they love. They are not making it clear to themselves that they can moderately eat foodstuff which they like and cannot completely give up.

This is why many people are totally against dieting as they confuse the term with starving themselves.

People should know that if a diet plan they adopt has to be successful, then they have to change their view on the food they prefer eating and must compromise with their personal likes for a certain period of time. Again, one more thing which people do not seem to understand is that food is not our enemy, but our inability to correctly divide and consume it is.

Very often, most of the population ends up eating the wrong foods more than the correct foods which ought to be consumed. This is the epicenter of the problem.

Five portions of veggies and three of fruits are the right amount of food that we must consume every day for getting the right q uantity of nutrients necessary. If this is not fulfilled, we tend to feel deprived and suffer hunger pangs. If we correctly consume the above-mentioned servings of fruits and vegetables, we are unlikely to have freq uent hunger pangs.

This implies we can enjoy the food we love in moderation as it has to be. The size per serving is another major problem. We are so used to eat the extra large pack of fries and the large cup of colas and other beverages that we fail to understand what the correct serving size is. All such temptations must be avoided and only what is needed must be consumed.

We must make it a point to always remember that dieting is not starving and hence must feel good about the whole process and motivate ourselves to take it up.

All the positive aspects of dieting and weight loss must be kept in mind always, rather than feeling low about the excess weight you are carrying with you now.

A positive outlook on the whole thing is to be adopted and you must keep motivating yourself even if the process of losing weight is taking longer than expected. Keep telling it to yourself that you would be getting your youthful body back.

However, dieting does not mean you should completely stop enjoying things which you liked. You can treat yourself to some goodies once in a while in moderation. After this, for burning the extra calories that you have consumed choose an activity which you cherish and enjoy.

This way, you get double the benefit. The exercises you have taken up must be something which you look forward to and enjoy. This would help in achieving better results. To be a successful dieter, you need to be confident and have a positive approach towards the whole dieting program. If you cannot keep yourself away in case of indulging, then it is better to avoid indulging, however, though it may be.

Nonetheless, if you are happy and feel good about the whole concept of dieting and exercise and keeping fit, then having little treats in moderation once in a while is a great option.

Chapter 4

------ ❧❧❧❧ ------

How to Benefit from Low-Calorie Diets

Low-calorie diets are probably the most basic of all diet plans. In most cases, they are straightforward and right to the point.

The premise of them is that if you reduce the number of calories that you take in on a daily basis, and continue the same level of activity, you will lose weight. Over the years, low-calorie diets have been proven to work, and to work well. But, if this is the case, then why is it that there are so many different diets on the market?

The reality is that most diets are simply different variations of the same idea dressed up for different purposes, mainly to sell books, or dieting plans, or fat burning pills or eq uipment. Some of these different dieting books are helpful in that they provide healthy recipes and they point out healthy food choices that you can make to help you lose weight.

They can also provide you with a structure and some motivation in the way of mapping out a plan and providing a series of success stories about other people who have overcome obesity by following that plan.

If you feel that you need that extra support, then there is nothing wrong with buying a book and following a plan like the one you are reading.

But, what happens more often than not is that people are looking for the "silver bullet" of low-calorie diets that will make them lose weight with very little effort on their part.

As a result, as soon as the dieting plan laid out looks like work, they start looking for the newest, latest and greatest diet that promises to tell them the fat burning secrets of the century. It is this attitude that the whole dieting industry thrives on, and is one of the reasons that people are gaining more weight and there is more obesity than ever in a country that has more dieting resources than ever before.

The bottom line is that a successful diet plan works when using low-calorie diets to make good health choices. If you want to reach a healthy weight, you need to increase the amount of healthy food you consume and reduce the number of overall calorie intake in.

Eliminating sugary foods and replacing fatty food with low-fat foods can make a big difference and will help you lose fat. Increasing the fat burning activities you do on a daily basis will also help. In reality, the choice is completely yours about how you want to view and use low-calorie diets.

Choose now to make small changes on a daily basis. Don't go overboard and try to starve yourself. Look for healthy recipes, eat fresh and whole foods, drink lots of water and move your body. With these small changes you will feel better in no time and soon you will also lose weight.

TIPS TO STICKING TO YOUR LOW-CALORIE DIET

Here you can find tips to help you fight the hunger during a short, low-calorie diet and lose the weight you wanted to.

1.   CHOOSE A DIET PLAN YOU LIKE

The idea behind most of the low-calorie diets is the same, so it does not really matter which diet plan you choose. So, pick the one which has the foods you like. If you hate cabbage, it does not make much sense to try to stay on the cabbage soup diet for a week takes a whole month.

2.   FIGURE OUT THE BEST TIME TO DIET

The holiday season, a lot of stress at work or special occasions make it harder to follow your diet. Look at your agenda and choose a time period when there is not much happening.

3.   BELIEVE IN YOURSELF

If you doubt your ability to go through the whole diet without relapses, you will set yourself up for failure.

If you think you will most likely end up eating candy during the diet anyway, you might as well not do it at all since a thought like that is almost like permitting yourself to break the diet.

4.   GET READY FOR POSSIBLE DIFFICULTIES

Take a moment to think about the challenges you will face during the diet. What is your biggest problem when it comes to dieting? Will you have to face difficult situations during the diet?

Now, think about how you will solve the problem or what will you do in the situation if it arises. It is much easier to stick to your diet if you have a well-thought strategy for dealing with the problem.

5. DO NOT TEST YOUR WILLPOWER UNNECESSARILY

It is easier to stick to your diet if you get rid of all the threats you might have in the house before starting the diet. Also, make a shopping list and buy everything you need for the diet at once.

Do not go shopping during the diet. If you absolutely have to go to the grocery while dieting, make a shopping list at home and decide not to buy anything, I mean anything which is not listed there. Do not even go to the nails where they sell the foods you want to avoid.

6. FIND SOMETHING TO DO

Play with the kids. Go to the opera. Do a jigsaw puzzle or some gardening. Fix the broken jacket. Anything to keep yourself busy! If you have a lot of free time, you will start thinking about food.

7. GET SOME SUPPORT

Talk about your diet to your family and friends and ask for their support. Perhaps someone would be willing to start the diet with you? However, if you do not feel comfortable about sharing the dieting with anyone you know, there are many online communities full of nice people willing to help you and share your experience with you.

8.   NO CHEATING

This diet is for you, for just 30 days, so cheating on the diet means cheating on yourself and will make your hard efforts useless.

Stick to the diet! If you are worried about your ability to follow the diet, you can start a food diary to write down what you have eaten during the day and give both the diet plan and your food diary to someone you trust after every diet day.

Chapter 5

─ ─ ─ ─ ─ ❧☙❧☙ ─ ─ ─ ─ ─

Healthy Diet Plans

Many people falsely believe that their lack of good health is a result of bad genetics or simply bad luck.

Actually, you have almost complete control over our health, and it's through eating healthy diet plans. Believe it or not, the foods you put into your body are almost entirely responsible for your overall health and fitness state.

Good eating habits can overcome bad genetics and luck anytime. Here are some tips to get you on the right track to eating healthy foods and living a long and healthy life.

First of all, increase your consumption of raw foods. Raw foods are any foods that have enzymes in them to aid in digestion. Try to make sure you consume at least 75% of your foods raw.

Here are the foods you should be primarily focusing on: fruits, vegetables, nuts, seeds, legumes, and sprouts. These foods will help you live a long and healthy life. The reason they are so good for you is that they all come from the plant.

How natural is it to consume an animal that has been living in extremely cramped q uarters its' whole life and has been fed large amounts of food to increase their body fat so they provide more meat? Does this strike you as a natural way to eat and stay healthy?

On the contrast, some of the healthiest and longest living civilization in the world consume primarily raw foods. Believe it or not, despite what you've heard about not being able to obtain enough protein and other essential elements through plant foods, they actually provide every essential vitamin and mineral your body needs to stay healthy. Take protein, for instance.

A common myth is that you can't get enough protein through plant food. Actually, there are many different excellent protein sources provided by raw foods. Great examples would be carrots and especially raw nuts.

Make sure, however, that you soak your nuts before consuming them raw. Raw and unsoaked nuts contain enzyme inhibitors that, when you eat them, will make you feel tired.

Soaking the nuts releases theses enzymes and allows you to enjoy soaked nuts and feel great as a result.

The bottom line: your health is in your hands. It is not up to luck, fate, or genetics it is up to you. If these healthy diet plans seem overwhelming to you, don't attempt to change your whole diet overnight; take your time. Try eating one healthy meal a week, and gradually increase that number two, three, till you reach a whole month target.

The more you consume these natural foods, the better you will feel, and the more motivate you will be to eating this way. Follow these healthy diet plans, and watch your overall health, happiness, and q uality of life skyrocket faster than you ever thought possible.

Chapter 6

_____ ❧❧❧ _____

Why Natural Diets can Fail; Especially Whole Diet Plan

Many people subscribe to fad diet plans that boost the income sheets of companies while leaving dieters in the lurch when it comes to their long-term health. Fortunately, though, there are things you can do to take matters into your own hands.

Once you have settled on a natural diet plan, avoid the following mistakes, and your effort will bear fruit.

1.   Poor planning: Many people start out with big ideas about what they are capable of but soon find that they were overambitious. A good plan should have the long-term picture in mind, meaning that your day-to-day life should not be too difficult.

The plan should involve small, doable steps that easily integrate into your life. The fastest way to undermine yourself is to assign yourself too much exercise or make your diet plan too restrictive.

2. Going it alone: There are all sorts of evidence showing that people who diet with other people, especially people they live with or with whom they are otherwise close, have a much higher success rate than those who attempt to go it alone.

There is strength in teamwork, and there is also the fact that dieting with partners or as a team gives you someone to whom you are accountable, which can be a powerful motivating factor.

3. Expecting it to work too fast: Any sane diet plan will enact minor changes to your life aimed at helping you not only be healthy, but also lose a little bit of weight on a week-by-week for a month scale. If you are doing things right, then there might not be a noticeable change in your weight for multiple weeks (unless you have one of those high-tech scales that measures you in ounces).

If you go into it thinking you are going to shed all your excess weight by the end of the month, then it is probably not going to stick.

4.   Allowing too many exceptions: A diet plan should truly be carefully thought-out plan that you actually stick to and then sticking to it is the most important part.

Embrace the structure that a diet plan gives to your life, and reject anything that takes you out of this structure.

5.   Giving up too easily: For many people in the throes of a difficult diet, a couple of lapses can seem like game over. There is a tendency to think that if you fail in a day or two, then the whole diet is a failure. But it does not have to be like that at all.

Any time you lapse in your diet plan, just remember all the progress you have made and remember that even with your lapses you are still better off than you were when you started out. You can always start fresh.

Chapter 7

———— ❧❧❧ ————

Diet and Nutrition is All About Good Common Sense

When you think about diet and nutrition do you imagine something harsh and rigid? Some kind of a diet that you will not be able to do, come what may? Perhaps, even something that is distasteful to you? Whatever made you think that? In reality, a diet and nutrition plan is quite far from any harsh action plan or crash course that you may have thought of.

You must be thinking that you have to cut down on your favorite foodstuff and maybe you also need to spend an exorbitant sum of money on a dietician.

The truth is, as far as your diet and nutrition goals, it is even simpler to put into action than you can ever imagine. In fact, you will be surprised to learn that all you need is some common sense.

Just about anyone can have a diet that is healthy, something which is real good for the body. It does not mean you have to change your whole diet or start starving yourself.

All you need to do is add foods to your diet that have all the necessary ingredients to keep you fit and fine. Perhaps, a greater need for you will be in cutting down on your intake of fatty foods, sugar, and salt. There is no secret recipe or a great mystery that is involved in a good diet or you have food that is nutritious every day.

You can get all the nutrition you want and be on a great diet as well just by eating simple foods like vegetables and fruits, every day. You should have foods that also have great starch content as well as foodstuffs that contain a good deal of protein.

One thing very important for you, as part of your plan to have a healthy and nutritious diet, is to drink a lot of water every day, all through the day. In fact, you should drink around one and a half liters of water a day, without fail.

Once you come to a proper understanding that you do not have to follow some kind of rigorous routine or that there is no need to restrict yourself to consuming just certain kinds of foods which you might find distasteful, you will find that you too can have a proper diet and nutrition, and enjoy the benefits of a healthy and a beautiful body and mind.

Chapter 8

─────── ❧❧❧❧ ───────

Whole Diet; What is the Whole Diet All About?

So just what is the Whole diet and what exactly is it all about?

Thanks to the obscene levels of obesity and rife levels of heart disease and diabetes, there has never been a greater focus on the overall society to become fit, slimmer and healthier.

Dieting and nutritional lifestyle choices have become endless and it would be fair to say that dieting in one way or another is now a way of life for the majority of people. And there are so, so many diets and programs available to us these days.

They cover every topic known to man on the right foods to eat and avoid and in what combination, but really, upon searching deeper, we will find that the answers we seek go back to our caveman ancestors. With this endless choice and all the varying options and rules involved in each particular diet, it pays to really understand what each diet entails before you choose one and get started.

It must be right for you and give you everything you need or are looking for without causing any additional problems or side effects.

Upon investigation, you will see that many popular diets restrict carbohydrates or focus on fruit and vegetables. Other diets focus on only eating a certain food group or even raw foods only.

Several also restrict or discourage large amounts of protein and meats. The Paleo Diet is q uite uniq ue, however, because the whole idea comes from simulating the natural aspects of the type of diet enjoyed by the very first humans - the caveman! What Is The Paleo Diet?

WHAT IS THE WHOLE DIET AND WHERE DOES IT COME FROM?

Known commonly as The Stone Age, Paleo comes from the Paleolithic period of history and the Paleo diet eating plan is often known as the "Hunter-Gatherer Diet." It takes its name from the fact that all the food contained in this diet were either able to be hunted or gathered. Meats and Seafood come under the hunted category, meanwhile, nuts, vegetables, and fruits, for example, are categorized under gathered.

Basically, this diet stems from the fact that early humans who had no access to or knowledge of animal husbandry and agriculture, had a diet that you either hunted or gathered for yourself.

The Whole diet applies this slant and line of thinking to modern-day foods, reducing and eliminating processed and man-made foods. This does not mean you are expected to hunt and gather for yourself! Just only that the nutrition choices we make are as natural and unaltered as possible. The base foundation of the Paleo eating plan is that humans are genetically suited to eat the foods that our ancestors consumed.

Therefore, before the introduction of agriculture, nutrition and food were so much different than that of today, so in short, the WHOLE DIET imitates the foods that every single human on earth consumed and had available at that particular time.

Not only is the Whole eating plan full of quality, natural, high nutritional value foods such as fruits and vegetables along with seafood and lean meats, but it is perhaps known best for the foods, drinks, and ingredients that are not consumed by those on the Whole Diet.

As the agriculture revolution provided us with foods our early ancestors never had, such as dairy products, salt, sugar, and even grains, they are not allowed to be consumed.

Not only do some of these ingredients and foodstuffs cause digestive problems, but these products have been shown through endless research that they can lead to an increase in weight and a higher chance of developing health problems such as diabetes.

Because of its high protein content, the Paleo nutritional lifestyle has a large and steadily growing athlete following. Thanks to the basic foods in the Paleo diet such as chicken, fish, lean meats, nuts, fruits and vegetables it is an athlete's dream providing energy, muscle development, and fiber along with the reduction of all weights gaining and physiq ue robbing junk food and unhelpful ingredients.

Most vegetables are great for the Whole lifestyle, however, root vegetables will give you the biggest bang for your buck health wise. One of the most basic reasons why the Paleo diet lifestyle is healthy for you is simply because you practically reduce all additives and artificial preservatives, many of which have been proven to be harmful to your health.

So that's the basic premise, which hopefully answers your q uestion, What is the Paleo diet eating plan all about yet you may still be q uestioning why you would make the significant switch to the Paleo Diet.

There are many health benefits associated with this diet and not the least of them is a potential relief for allergy sufferers thanks to the fact that the Whole Diet is naturally allergen free.

Two of the biggest causes of common allergies, gluten, and casein, are commonly found in manufacturing foods. Because the overwhelming majority of foods available on the Paleo diet do not contain either gluten or casein, allergy sufferers can rejoice!

But don't forget about the weight loss potential for those on the Paleo. Apart from the protein aspect which is great for weight loss alone, the Paleo diet is naturally low in carbohydrates and has a low caloric count. It is also naturally high in fiber, which is a crucial factor when it comes to overeating and weight loss.

The low carbohydrates combined with the high amounts of natural fiber while on this diet ensures that the risk of coronary heart disease, diabetes and other weight-related illnesses and ailments is decreased.

Last but not least, this diet has none of the other big risks when it comes to heart disease and cancer like additives, sugar, salt, saturated fats and of course the big one getting a heap of exposure in recent years, hydrogenated oils or trans fats as they are commonly known.

At first glance, the Paleo Diet, lifestyle can seem like a hard choice to make with limited food options, however, if you look closer and explore a little deeper, those fears will be addressed and upon making some small worthy sacrifices you will be bettering your chance of actually living a healthier and happier, disease free life! And just remember that as close as you can get to this lifestyle choice, the benefits will start to appear.

Like as in exercise, 5 sit-ups is better than zero and going for a 20-minute walk is better than sitting on the couch! Same thing goes for the Whole Diet! Although following the diet 100% is ideal, your body will still start to thank you for every single step you take on living the ideals of the Paleo Diet.

HOW TO INCORPORATE THE WHOLE DIET INTO YOUR LIFESTYLE

While there is no single way to get started on a Whole Diet, there are many wrong ways. Because of Whole's balanced approach to nutrition, many people embrace the whole Whole lifestyle as a way to lose weight. But being able to, incorporate it successfully can be challenging, especially for Paleo newcomers.

The foundation of the Paleo philosophy is built on eliminating processed foods from your diet because our ancestors did not have these types of foods. As a general rule of thumb, if a food item is pre-made, don't eat it. Meat, fresh fruit and vegetables, eggs, nuts, and healthy oils such as olive oil are foods that you can eat on this diet. Creating well-balanced meals can be difficult.

BREAKFAST EXAMPLES

Since eggs are rich in protein and low in calories, many people on the Paleo Diet incorporate them into breakfast. Poached eggs with olive oil and sea salt, fruit salad and low-calorie omelette with spinach and mushrooms are all Whole Diet friendly meals that you can enjoy on this diet.

Since dairy is not allowed, you should not use milk or cheese. However, almond milk is a great alternative that works with this diet.

LUNCH EXAMPLES

For lunch, you can enjoy a large, fresh tossed salad with olive oil and vinegar for dressing and a few nuts for added protein. You can also incorporate meat into your lunch, such as grilled chicken with vegetables or salsa.

DINNER EXAMPLES

Dinner meal ideas are similar to lunch since many people like to incorporate meat and veggies into their entree. Fish and steamed broccoli, chicken stir fry, and steak are all acceptable meals on the Paleo Diet.

Salmon and other seafood meals are also options to consider. However, you should be careful with how you prepare your meals. Never fry or bread, meat. Most carbohydrates such as bread are not allowed on the Whole Diet. You can bake, broil, grill and even boil meat as a healthier alternative.

SNACKS

Snack time can be challenging while on the Paleo Diet. Keep fresh fruit and nuts on hand to avoid giving in to temptation snack foods. You can also prepare your own fresh vegetable tray with an olive oil based dipping sauce. Fruit salad is another popular snack food in the Whole Diet.

If you prefer a meat-based snack, you can create a q uick and healthy snack wrap. Simply place lunch meat and your favorite sandwich, veggies in a large lettuce leaf, wrap, and enjoy.

COUNTING CALORIES

Most people on the Paleo Diet do not count their calories. However, if you are committed to losing weight you should keep track of your calories. Since the Paleo Diet can be low carb, depending on which foods you eat the most, it is important to speak with your doctor before starting it to ensure that it is right for you. The WHOLE DIET is essentially a type of low carb diet.

It can help you lose those stubborn pounds and develop the muscle definition you have been dreaming of. Get started with these meal ideas.

IS THE WHOLE DIET SAFE?

As with any new, or newly popular, diet, it has become common for people to question whether the Whole Diet is safe.

The Whole Diet is, of course, a way of eating based on the diet of Paleolithic Man, the hunter-gatherer, or caveman. So what is the answer? Are we right to q uestion it, and is the Paleo Diet safe or is it just another potentially dangerous fad?

LOW CARBOHYDRATE DIETS

The first possible objection to the Whole way of eating is based largely on a misconception, the idea that it is a low carb diet. The Whole Diet certainly shares some similarities with the well know, and perhaps infamous, Atkins Diet.

Like Atkins, Whole Diet suggests high fat and protein intake and includes far fewer carbohydrates than we are generally used to eating.

Unlike the Atkins diet, however, the WHOLE DIET does not seek to restrict carbohydrate intake, and it is that extreme restriction that can cause problems and, potentially, be dangerous. If you deliberately, and greatly, restrict your carbohydrate intake in order to remain in ketosis, the major aim of the Atkins diet and its process of weight loss, then you really do need to be careful.

This method, if attempted at all, is probably best supervised by a medical professional, it can certainly produce some side effects that are unpleasant. This is not to say that it's not effective, for it does seem to get results, but there's really nothing to suggest that this is how we are naturally meant to eat.

So, rather than being deliberately low in carbohydrates, the Whole Diet just tends to be so because it removes grains, sugars, and potatoes, the major sources of carbohydrate in most people's diets. When you take those staple foods out of the eq uation, most people who try the Paleo diet find themselves looking for ways to get more carbohydrates, not restrict their intake. But is the Paleo diet safe in terms of this lower carbohydrate intake?

Yes, because it is a diet based on a balance of nutritionally rich foods, not on the idea of restriction.

HIGH-FAT DIETS

The other major objection to the Paleo Diet, on medical grounds, is the encouragement to eat lots of protein and fats. The concern, of course, is the increase in cholesterol and the idea that eating all that fat is going to cause you to gain weight.

This is, however, not true. The capitalization is entirely justified as this is such a major, and yet common, mistake! There is research, and plenty of it, though far beyond the scope of this book, to show that it is not eating fats that cause you to gain weight but carbohydrates.

Refined sugars and grains, wheat, in particular, are the worst offenders here. As ever, it's best to do your own research, but you won't need to look far to find plenty of evidence that eating fat and protein, and plenty of it, is a good thing; it's certainly not the reason that people put on weight.

This shouldn't be taken as carte blanche on fatty foods - they're not all good, but the ones that are may come of something of a surprise. Again, it's beyond the scope of this book, but let's just say: butter, eggs, and fats from pastured, grass fed animals are all very good for you. But beware those vegetable oils - if you have to do any more than sq ueezing something to get the oil out of it, be suspicious! So, olive oil is well; corn, palm and soy oils are not.

The Wikipedia pages for those oils make for some interesting reading - you might want to learn more before putting any more of those in your body!

SO ARE THE WHOLE DIET SAFE OR NOT?

It does seem a little ironic that people will question the wisdom of something like the Whole Diet but happily continue eating refined sugars, modified starches and hexane extracted, hydrogenated oils that really have no place in the food-chain of any animal, let alone on human plates. And yet, of course, there is the illusion of safety in the known. It's true to say that Westerners in general, and Americans in particular, are more overweight and less healthy than has been the case for many decades, if ever.

Should you be tempted to q uestion this just take a look at some of the magazine advertisements and posters from the

1950s - skinny, not fat, was considered to be a problem in those days! So, rather than asking 'is the Whole Diet safe?', you might, perhaps, be wondering how safe your current diet is.

The Paleo Diet is one based on natural balance. It's a very different balance than the one we've been taught for years, but it is balanced, it is not a diet of extremes.

You should view with suspicion any diet that calls for extreme actions, especially if it involves restricting certain food groups, such as carbohydrates or fats. Nature loves balance, and will generally have it one way or another.

So, are you still asking Is the Paleo Diet Safe? Perhaps the best answer is simply to try it for yourself. When you notice how good you start to feel, how weight naturally drops off if you need it to, and how much energy and vitality you have, there will be a clue.

If you see skin conditions, aches and pains and digestive problems disappearing, then you may well be asking not whether the Whole Diet is safe but why you didn't get around to trying it sooner.

EVERYDAY WHOLE DIET RECIPES

Well, being and fitness nuts and exercise buffs browsing for a long in addition to easy-to-follow diet should find that the Paleo food regimen will be one of the finest selections to a more healthy life, plus Paleo diet meal plans are on the list of best-tasting healthy foods ever.

In place of trying to approach being on a diet being an endeavor that restricts our affection for foodstuff and also takes away the tastiness of every dinner, you ought to go for a more natural and sustainable diet plan.

The majority of weight loss plans fails due to individuals feel unfulfilled with regards to below passable effects, or they comprehend they cannot sustain the req uirements of the food plan during lengthy time periods.

EASY COOKING FOR WHOLE DIET RECIPES

As such, why the Whole food plan had been brought to the fore. Your best choice to preserve your req uired body weight and also improve our strength plus stamina is to devour similar foodstuffs which our historic predecessors feasted upon.

The situation with the latest diet fads is since will not give you varieties of food choices to include in your food. On the other hand, diet recipes of Paleo let you mix and match your favorite meats, vegetables and also ingredients to produce the ideal Paleo meal. The best thing with regards to being on a diet the Paleolithic manner is the fact you can tailor your meals freely and enjoy meals that you just like the most.

There is, of course, a number of restrictions, namely keeping clear of processed foods and from sweets, but this really is just similar to how any other diet programs.

In fact, this diet recipe is fashioned to comply to the taste buds of individuals. Ingesting like our hunter-gatherer ancestors will not mean that you should devour raw meat and raw vegetables.

What the Paleo guides you through is known as a back-to-basics mentality we should eat only the things which are good for the health and wellness and discount everything else.

WHOLE DIET RECIPES FOR GOOD NUTRITIONAL CONSUMPTION

The linchpin of the diet is facilitating nutritional consumption through every last meal that we eat. We throw out processed, salty and sweet cuisine basically because they include absolutely no nutritive value anyway, and may even result in critical health problems over time.

However, there is no need to compromise taste and visual passion for the sake of nutritional consumption. Diet recipes are usually not over zealous or exotic meals which may only be cooked through unique ways and fancy eq uipment.

In truth, the food preparation techniq ues which are used by our grandmothers could be the very same things that we need to learn as a way to cook dishes the Paleo way. That's the beauty of the diet recipes of Paleo.

CREATE YOUR WHOLE DIET GROCERY LIST

OK, then. Let's get shopping with your Whole Diet grocery list!

You're all fired up and ready to make a start on what just could be the most important nutritional decision in your life so far... commencing the Paleo Eating Plan! It really is a great decision and if you stick to it, a decision that will pay off in so many ways when it comes to losing weight, detoxing your system, avoiding food intolerance's and just feeling much healthier in general! Now you need a WHOLE DIET Grocery list for all those Paleo diet recipes.

I have separated the Whole Diet grocery list below into categories that start with foods your inner caveman absolutely craves and then gradually goes down the Whole pyramid until we end up at foods that you should definitely avoid and should never be in your Whole Diet shopping list.

Take notes, read this very good or better still, print this out, do whatever you have to do in order to ensure you have the best chance at making a successful conversion to the Paleo lifestyle and following the Paleo Diet Guidelines.

WHOLE DIET GROCERY LIST ESSENTIALS

Now just one more thing before we get started on some yummy Paleo diet meals. There are those who say that the Whole Diet menu is quite limited. As you will see just on the list below, this could not be further from the truth. Enjoy!

Looking at meats first; Whole Diet Grocery List

Beef, lean cuts only

Chuck steak

Hamburger, extra-lean (no more than 7 % fat).

Flank steak.

Lean pork, visible fat trimmed.

Pork chops and pork loin.

Top sirloin steak.

Lean veal.

You can also easily add most sorts of game meats to this category. The regular game meats such as venison, goose, and alligator are popular options, however, just about all game is acceptable from rattlesnake and pheasant to wild boar and reindeer. Just always remember to choose lean cuts with no fat.

Lean poultry is also a winner for your Whole Diet grocery list but ensures it is only the white meat parts, preferably only the breast portion and that the skin is removed.

The ocean provides those on the Whole Diet plan a wealth of meal choices! Nosh away on all of these tasty seafood options...

Bass, Bluefish, Cod, Drum, Eel.

Grouper, Haddock, Halibut, Herring.

Mackerel, Monk Fish, Mullet, Perch.

Northern Pike, Rockfish, Orange Roughly, Salmon.

Scrod, Shark, Red Snapper, Sunfish.

Tilapia, Trout, Tuna, Turbot and Walleye.

Shellfish is on the Paleo diet grocery list too!

Abalone, Clams, Crab, Crayfish.

Lobster, Mussels, Oysters, Scallops and shrimps (prawns).

Of course, there are still q uite a few species of both fish and shellfish that I haven't included on this list but I'm sure you get the drift...

Chicken, duck and goose eggs are also great, however, please only limit yourself to a maximum of 6 eggs per week!

Whole Diet Grocery List Items From The Fruit And Vegetable Department.

As you would imagine, fruit and veggies make up a huge part of the Whole lifestyle and should make up a large portion of your Whole Diet grocery list! These are the best of the bunch; get into them.

Apple, Apricot, Avocado, Banana, Blackberries, Blueberries, Boysenberries, Cantaloupe, Chermoya, Cherries, Cranberries, Figs, Gooseberries, Grapefruit, Grapes, Guava, Kiwi, Lemon, Lychee, Mango, Cassava melon, Honeydew melon, Nectarine, Orange, PapPaleo Diet Grocery Listaya, Passion fruit, Peaches, Pears, Persimmon, Pineapple, Plum, Pomegranate, Rhubarb, Starfruit, Strawberries, Tangerine, Watermelon. You just can't go wrong with any of those!

And now, heading over to the vegetable section; stock your crisper and refrigerators with these healthy Paleo choices. Artichoke, Asparagus, Beet greens, Broccoli, Brussels spouts,

Cabbage, Carrots, Cauliflower, Celery, Collards, Cucumber and Bell peppers.

Seeds and nuts are also an extremely good resource, they taste great and are very filling! Try to eat as many of these varieties as you can and ensure most of them are regulars on your Paleo diet grocery list.

Almonds, Brazil nuts, Cashews, Chestnuts, Hazelnuts, Macadamia nuts, Pecans, Pine nuts, Pistachios (unsalted), Pumpkin seeds, Sesame seeds, Sunflower seeds, Walnuts.

All of the foods listed above are perfectly Paleo approved meals and should form the bulk of your Paleo Diet shopping list. There are absolutely loads of choices available and definitely more than enough variety to keep you happy! Go nuts with all of them.

WHOLE DIET GROCERY LIST MODERATION ITEMS.

Now the list of foods below is all Paleo approved, however, they are not as good as the ones listed above. They can be enjoyed, however, only in moderation. Try and limit their intake just to treat foods or that something different now and then.

For the oil lovers out there, any of these Avocado, Olive, Flaxseed, Walnut and Canola are acceptable, however, try and limit yourself to only 4 tablespoons maximum per day.

OK, so our cavemen ancestors didn't have beer, wine or spirits after a tough day, but most Paleo diet plan convert is allowed to indulge just a little bit! Coffee and Tea are also OK in moderation and also soda, however, make sure it is the diet or sugar-free variety.

On the sweet side; well that is probably the only area where critics of the Paleo diet eating plan have some grounding. There aren't a whole lot of sweets and desserts that you can have on your Paleo diet grocery list.

The good thing is that after getting used to this way of eating, you really won't crave the sweet stuff as much as you used to and when you start to feel so much better; well; it's an easy tradeoff.

Another good thing is that few people really eat a good variety of fresh fruit. Apples, oranges, bananas and grapes make up most of the fruit that gets eaten. There is a whole sweet spectrum of taste, texture, smells and variety of fresh fruit and once you realize this; you will find that the sweet cravings you used to have for cakes and candy are gone!

Get Shopping!

When you first start out on the Paleo diet eating plan it can seem tough to get your head around and be sure of what you can eat. I hope that this chapter has helped explain what items are the best and should always be staples on your Paleo Diet Grocery List.

When first starting out with the Paleo lifestyle it may seem like your choices for meals are limited. However the closer you look and the deeper you dig, you will q uickly see that there are countless options to live Paleo and they are not all bland and boring either.

Chapter 9

Whole Diet

Whole Diet is all about cutting out foods that might be having a negative impact on your health.

Now, what you can eat?

Whole Diet can be as simple as you want it to be. Despite the huge collection of amazing Whole recipes, you don't need to make it complicated if you don't want to.

Your Whole Diet grocery list can be as simple as:

- Meat
- Vegetables
- Fruit

1.   PROTEIN (MEAT AND EGGS)

You'll be eating massive amounts of protein during Whole Diet, so it's time to stock up!

Grass-Fed Beef

Organic/Pastured Chicken and Pork

Wild-Caught Fish

In an ideal world, you'll purchase grass-fed, organic, and pastured meat. If you can't afford it, no worries; just buy the leanest cuts you can and trim the fat and skin before eating. Commercially raised, processed meats are not permitted (no bacon, sausage, or deli meats.

2.   VEGETABLES

Veggies are tasty and good for you! Good thing, because you'll be eating a lot of them. Aim for local and seasonal veggies, which will be the most affordable (with more nutrients too). Remember, frozen veggies are a solid option.

They often cost less, can keep for longer in the freezer, and sometimes are more nutritious than fresh produce counterparts.

While frozen vegetables are flash-frozen right after being harvested, regular fresh grocery produce spends days (or longer) in cooler trucks being shipped to grocery stores, making them, oddly enough, not as fresh as the frozen stuff. All veggies are allowed on Whole Diet except corn, peas, and lima beans.

Some vegetable suggestions for the Whole food list include:

Broccoli

Brussels Sprouts

Butternut Sq uash (try it with this butternut sq uash lasagna recipe)

Spaghetti Sq uash (great for imitation noodles)

Carrots

Cauliflower (perfect for cauliflower rice)

Eggplant

Kale

Lettuce (for salads of course)

Mushrooms

Onion

Potatoes (yup, they're allowed)

Spinach

Summer Sq uash

Tomatoes

Yams

Zucchini

3.   **FRUIT**

When it comes to fruit, organic and/or local fruits are best. Frozen fruit is a fine second option, don't be afraid to stock up on fruit as a sweet-tooth substitute.

All fruit is good to go on Whole Diet.

Some fruit suggestions for the Whole food list include:

Apples

Berries

Bananas

Cherries (these are my favorite Whole Diet desert)

Figs (grab a pack of Trader Joe's Turkish Figs – they taste just like Fig Newton's!)

Grapes

Grapefruit (great with morning eggs)

Lemons and Limes (you'll find them a lot in recipes)

Pineapple

4.   FATS

Good fats are another important component of your Whole Diet shopping list. Healthy fats will keep you full and will serve as a base for your Whole Diet meals. Some popular Whole healthy fats include:

Coconut milk

Avocados

Coconut Oil

Olive Oil

Organic ghee

Raw nuts

With your nuts and trail mixes, be sure to check your labels! You'd be shocked at how many naughty additives and sugars are slipped into nut packs.

If you're looking to cook some great Whole-friendly dishes, you may want to make a point to pick up these ingredients, which are common in the most popular Whole Diet recipes:

1.   Coconut Oil. We talked about this earlier, but it's worth spending a few more words on. Coconut oil is the most prominent ingredient in Whole Diet recipes; you'll find it listed absolutely everywhere. It's a tasty, healthy cooking oil Whole folks can't get enough of! You'll definitely need to include this on your Whole Diet shopping list.

2.   Ghee. This is another ingredient you'll see everywhere for Whole recipes. Ghee is clarified butter, which is basically butter without the milk solids.

3.   Almond/Coconut Flour. Great for breading your meats or for thickening sauces. Use coconut flour with this buffalo chicken fingers recipe which is one of my favorites Whole Diet recipes.

4.   Apple Cider Vinegar. Apple cider vinegar is an ingredient in many sauces and salad dressing recipes.

5.   Mustard. Mustard is one of the few toppings you can buy safely at the store (still, make sure to check the labels). It's good to have handy for burger nights.

6.   Coconut Aminos: Used in many tasty recipes for sauces. If you're lucky you'll find it at a health food store, or you can grab it online.

Chapter 10

------ ❧❧❧ ------

Delicious Whole Dinner Recipes

POULTRY

1.   THAI CHICKEN WITH SPICY "PEANUT" SAUCE

A Thai-inspired stir-fry sounds innocent enough (veggies! meat! dairy-free!), but it can be a minefield of Whole Diet no-no's, such as soy sauce, honey, and peanut butter. This recipe gets around those roadblocks, subbing in coconut amino's for the soy, a mashed date for sweetness, and sunflower butter as a vitamin E-rich replacement for the peanutty stuff.

INGREDIENTS

1 date

Water

1 garlic clove, pressed

1 T fresh ginger, finely grated

¼ C sunflower butter

Juice of ½ lime

4 T coconut amino

1 T sesame oil

⅛ tsp salt

Red pepper flakes

4 T olive oil

1 lb. chicken tenders

Salt

Pepper

2 medium zucchinis, spiralized

1 handful of carrot shreds

2 sweet peppers, thinly sliced

Sesame seeds

Cilantro, chopped

INSTRUCTIONS

1.   Put the date in a small cup and add enough water to complete cover date. Microwave on high for 1 minute and allow to soak until the date is needed later.

2.   In a small bowl, whisk together garlic, ginger, sunflower butter, lime juice, coconut amino, sesame oil, and salt.

3.   Remove date from the water. Cut pits out of date and discard. With a fork, smash date until it turns into a paste. Whisk date pastes with the rest of the "peanut" sauce.

4.   Add a dash of red pepper flakes to the sauce, enough to add as much heat as preferred.

5.   In a skillet warm 2 T of olive oil over medium-high heat. Add chicken tenders and sauté on each side for 3-4 minutes or until cooked thoroughly. Remove chicken from skillet and set aside to rest and cool.

6.   In the same skillet, add the remaining 2 T of olive oil. Toss zucchini, carrot shreds and sweet peppers in the oil. Stir constantly with tongs and allow to cook for 2 minutes, just long enough to warm the vegetables thoroughly and slightly soften.

7.   Dice chicken and toss with the veggie noodles. Stir in the sauce just before serving.

8.   Garnish with sesame seeds and cilantro.

2.   ROASTED LEMON CHICKEN WITH POTATOES AND ROSEMARY

Already a pretty clean meal, the classic chicken and potato dish didn't need too much tweaking to become Whole compliant. Translation: It's a great way to ease yourself into the plan. Just spruce up the protein with a spritz of lemon and the carbs with garlic and rosemary. You've got a succulent dinner that'll make you forget you gave up anything at all.

INGREDIENTS

8-10 pieces of your favorite cut of chicken - skin on bone in

1 lbs. baby red potatoes

1/2 in onion - cut large pieces

2 lemons 1 sliced and 1 juiced

1/3 cup olive oil

2 cloves garlic, minced

1 Tablespoon fresh Rosemary plus sprigs for garnish

1/2 teaspoon crushed red pepper flakes

1 1/2 teaspoon salt

1/2 teaspoon fresh ground pepper

INSTRUCTIONS

1.   Preheat oven to 400 degrees F.

2.   Spray a glass 13-in. x9-in. baking dish with cooking spray. Arrange chicken pieces (skin side up), potatoes, sliced onion and lemon slices evenly in pan.

3.   In a small bowl, whisk together lemon juice, olive oil, garlic, rosemary, crushed red pepper flakes, salt, and pepper.

4.   Pour mixture over chicken, making sure all the chicken is covered. Toss a bit if necessary.

5. Sprinkle generously with additional salt and pepper.

6. Bake uncovered for about 1 hour, or until chicken and potatoes are fully cooked.

3.   CHICKEN BALANCE BOWL

This fresh bowl has all our salad favorites; chicken, sweet potato, and avocado; and a sauce so good you'll want to make extra and keep it in the fridge. (Just double-check that the tahini you go with has no added sugar so it's Whole Diet approved.) A delicious dinner whipped up in 30 minutes?

INGREDIENTS

2 chicken thighs or breasts

12 Oz chopped Butternut sq uash (about 2 ½ cups)

1 tablespoon + 2 teaspoons coconut oil

6 cups mixed greens

1 avocado, chopped

¼ cup tahini

1 tablespoon lemon juice

1 tablespoon apple cider vinegar

3 tablespoons water

Salt

Pepper

Garlic powder

INSTRUCTIONS

1.   Preheat oven to 425 degrees. Place butternut sq uash on a baking sheet. Toss with 2 teaspoons of melted coconut oil, ½ teaspoon salt, ¼ teaspoon pepper & ¼ teaspoon garlic powder. Roast in the oven for 25 minutes, tossing around halfway through.

2.   Take your chicken and sprinkle both sides with salt, pepper and garlic powder. Place a large saute pan over medium-high heat. Add 1 tablespoon of coconut oil and let heat up for about 30 seconds. Then add chicken and cook for 3-4 minutes on each side, depending on how thick they are (If they are thick I suggest pounding them down a bit so they all have an even thickness). Set chicken aside.

3.   In a small bowl, combine tahini, lemon juice, apple cider vinegar, water, ½ teaspoon salt, ¼ teaspoon pepper & ¼ teaspoon garlic powder. Toss a couple of tablespoons of dressing over the greens in a large bowl until evenly coated.

4.   To assemble bowl, add lettuce and top with butternut squash, chopped chicken, and avocado pieces. Drizzle more tahini dressing on top and enjoy.

4. MANGO CHICKEN WITH COCONUT CAULIFLOWER RICE

This recipe makes two clever swaps: The first is cauliflower "rice" instead of the usual white grain, and the second is tapioca flour as breading for the chicken. Add ginger and trusty coconut amino's to round out this healthier version of a takeout classic. Genius.

INGREDIENTS

For the sauce:

2 1/2 tsp Coconut oil dividend

1 1/2 tsp Fresh ginger minced

1 tsp Garlic, minced

1/2 tsp Habanero pepper, minced

3/4 Cup Orange Mango or Mango, Juice (100% pure juice)

1/2 Tbsp Coconut amino

1 tsp Tapioca flour

For the chicken:

3 Tbsp Tapioca flour

8 oz Chicken breast patted dry and cut into one-inch cubes

Salt + Pepper

2 Tbsp Coconut Oil

For the cauliflower rice:

3 Cups Cauliflower, cut into bite-sized pieces

2 tsp Coconut oil

2 Tbsp Unsweetened coconut flakes

For garnish:

1/2 a Large mango, cut into cubes

Roughly chopped cilantro

Diced Green Onion

Toasted sesame seeds

INSTRUCTIONS

1.   In a medium pot over medium heat, melt 1 1/2 tsp of the coconut oil for the sauce. Add the ginger, garlic and Habanero pepper and cook until fragrant, about 1 minute.

2.   Add in the juice and coconut amino's. Raise the temperature to high heat and bring to a boil. Additionally, place the tapioca flour in a small bowl.

3.   Once the liq uid comes to a boil, add 2 tsp of it to the bowl with the tapioca flour and whisk until smooth. While stirring constantly, pour the tapioca mixture into the sauce and boil for 2 minutes.

4.   After the sauce as boiled, reduce the heat to medium-low and simmer, stirring frequently, until the sauce reduces by about 1/4 and becomes shiny about 6-7 minutes. Transfer to a large bowl to let it cool and thicken while you make the chicken.

5.   Place the tapioca flour into a large ziplock bag and season the cubed chicken with salt and pepper. Add the chicken in the bag and shake around until evenly coated with the flour.

6.   In a medium pan, heat 1 Tbsp of the coconut oil over medium-high heat. Place half of the chicken into the pan, being careful not to crowd it, and cook until golden brown, about 2-3 minutes. Flip and repeat. Transfer the chicken to a paper towel-lined plate and blot off an excess oil. Repeat with the remaining chicken. If the chicken starts cooking too fast, turn the heat down a little bit.

7.   While the chicken cooks, place the cauliflower into a large food processor and process until broken down and "rice-like"

8.   Heat the 2 tsp of coconut oil up in a large pan over medium-high heat and add the cauliflower and coconut flakes. Cook until light golden brown, about 2-3 minutes. Cover, reduce the heat to medium and cook until the cauliflower is tender about 2-4 minutes.

9.   Transfer the chicken and mango cubes into the bowl with the sauce and toss until evenly coated.

10.   Divide the chicken and cauliflower between two plates and garnish with cilantro, green onion, and sesame seeds.

This is also really good with just steamed cauliflower rice if you don't want to add the extra oil.

5.   JALAPENO TURKEY BURGER

With gluten, dairy, and even ketchup out of the picture, you've got to get creative to make burgers taste good. Here, guacamole, a poached egg, and jalapeños up the ante.

INGREDIENTS

1 pound ground turkey (I prefer 85% lean, it has more fat, which makes for a better burger!) If your ground turkey has excess liq uid, be sure to set on paper towels to remove the juices.

½-3/4 of one jalapeño pepper, minced

1 medium size shallot, peeled and minced

Zest and of one lime, and 2 teaspoon lime juice

2 Tablespoon chopped cilantro

1 teaspoon paprika

1 teaspoon cumin

½ a teaspoon sea salt

½ teaspoon black pepper

Guacamole

Pico de Gallo

Poached Egg (optional)

INSTRUCTIONS

1.   Note: The ground turkey to buy is the consistency of hamburger. If yours seems to have extra liq uid, set on paper towels to drain juices.

2.   Place turkey, herbs, spices and lime in a bowl and use hands to mix well.

3.   Form into four patties.

4.   Place pan on medium heat.

5.   Add olive oil to the bottom of the pan.

6.   When the pan is hot, place patties in pan and cook for about 5 minutes each side or until cooked through.

7.   Top with guacamole, Pico de Gallo, and poached egg if desired.

SEAFOOD

6.   GRILLED SALMON WITH MANGO SALSA

No restrictions on healthy fats while on the Whole Diet! And thank goodness for that, because we have a feeling you wouldn't be able to stay away from this cholesterol-slashing, omega-packed dish. Flaky salmon with a chunky mango salsa? Irresistible.

INGREDIENTS

4 6-ounce salmon fillets

1 teaspoon garlic powder

1 teaspoon chili powder

Salt and pepper to taste

Juice of 1 lime

Mango salsa

2-3 mangos, diced

½ red pepper,

½ red onion, diced

1 small jalapeño, seeded and finely chopped

¼ cup packed cilantro leaves, roughly chopped

INSTRUCTIONS

1.   In a medium bowl, stir together mangoes, red peppers, onions, jalapeños, and cilantro. Set aside until ready to use.

2.   Stir together garlic powder, chili powder, and salt and pepper (I used about a ½ teaspoon each). Rub mixture onto

salmon fillets. Grill over medium heat for 6-8 minutes on each side.

3.   Sq ueeze fresh lime juice over grilled salmon, then top with mango salsa and serve.

7.   WHITEFISH FILLET WITH BRAISED FENNEL

Not counting salt and pepper, there are only three ingredients in this dish. Plus the large fillet of white fish makes for a super-filling protein source. Pair it with fennel; the vitamin C-heavy cousin of carrots; for an easy but elegant dinner.

INGREDIENTS

White Fish Fillet

1 large white fish fillet per person

Pinch Himalayan or fine sea salt

Few grinds freshly cracked black pepper

The juice of half a lemon or lime

Braised Fennel

½ large fennel bulb per person

Pinch Himalayan or fine sea salt

Few grinds freshly cracked black pepper

INSTRUCTIONS

For the Braised Fennel

1.   Cut off the stalks from the fennel bulbs and cut each bulb lengthwise into 6 thick slices.

2.   It's important that you do not remove the core otherwise, the slices will fall apart.

3.   Season each fennel slice with a little bit of salt and pepper.

4.   In a large, heavy skillet, heat a little bit of olive oil or coconut oil over medium-high heat until your pan gets really hot. Add the fennel slices and cook until nice and brown, then flip the slices and cook the other side.

5.   Lower the heat, cover and continue cooking for about 6-8 minutes, until the fennel is good and tender.

For the fish fillets

1.   Pat the fish dry and season with a little bit of salt and pepper.

2.   Heat a little bit of olive or coconut oil in a medium non-stick skillet, over medium-high heat. When the pan is hot enough, add fillets and cook until it starts to form a little bit of a brown crust and flesh turns almost completely opaque. Very delicately flip the fillets and continue cooking until fish is cooked all the way through and no longer translucent. This should take about 1½ to 2 minutes per side, depending on thickness.

3.   Sprinkle with lemon or lime juice and transfer to dinner plates

4.   Serve with braised fennel, loaded coleslaw, and fresh greens.

8.   SHRIMP AND ASPARAGUS STIR-FRY

Coconut oil lends an appropriately tropical taste (not to mention antimicrobial benefits) to the shrimp in this light, brothy stir-fry. Simply seasoned with lemon, ginger, and garlic, it's the 15-minute clean meal you can throw together with no matter how tired you are after a busy day.

INGREDIENTS

2tablespoonscoconut oil

1poundshrimp, peeled

1bundleasparagus, chopped

2tablespoonslemon juice

4clovesgarlic, minced

1/2teaspoonground ginger

2/3cupbroth

INSTRUCTIONS

1.   Heat the fat in a skillet over medium-high heat.

2.   Add the shrimp, asparagus, lemon juice, garlic, and ginger to the pan.

3.   Cook about 2 minutes, then stir and cook another 2 minutes.

4.   Add the broth and simmer until the asparagus is tender and the shrimp is pink 2-4 minutes.

9.   BLACKENED CAJUN MAHI MAHI

This recipe calls for a few more spices than you might normally stock, but each will go a long way in flavoring the fish. And yes, you'll undoubtedly find yourself using them for other recipes while on the Whole Diet. Use them here for a rub to slather onto brain power-enhancing mahi-mahi fillets before the fish gets seared and topped with sliced avocado.

INGREDIENTS

Blacked Cajun Spice Rub

1 teaspoon dried parsley

1 teaspoon dried oregano

1 teaspoon dried thyme

1 teaspoon smoked paprika

½ teaspoon cayenne pepper*

½ teaspoon onion powder

½ teaspoon garlic powder

½ teaspoon salt

½ teaspoon pepper

Blackened Cajun Mahi Mahi

(2) 6oz wild caught Mahi filets, thawed and patted dry

1 tablespoon coconut oil

1 avocado, sliced

Lime wedges for serving

INSTRUCTIONS

1.   Make the spice rub by combining all the dried spices on a plate and stirring with a fork to combine.

2.   Heat a medium size skillet over medium-high heat. While it is heating up, dredge the fish fillets in the spice rub and coat evenly. When the pan is warm, add the coconut oil, and cook the spice-rubbed fish until cooked thru. Cooking time will depend on the thickness of your fish. Typically about 3 to 4 minutes per side.

3.   Serve warm. Top with sliced avocado and wedges of lime.

1/2 teaspoon cayenne pepper will make this mildly spicy. If you like it spicier, feel free to add more. If you are heat sensitive, add less or even leave it out so it is more kid friendly.

OTHER MEATS

10. SKILLET BEEF FAJITAS

This homey Tex-Mex favorite is packed with veggies and a spicy kick. Throw everything in a skillet, and you'll be done in 30 minutes. Just make sure your broth of choice is Whole Diet approved (or if you're game, make it from scratch).

INGREDIENTS

Steak:

1½ lb flank steak, sliced into thin ribbons against the grain

1 lime, juiced

½ teaspoon chili powder

¼ teaspoon of ground cayenne red pepper

⅛ teaspoon cumin

⅛ teaspoon paprika

⅛ teaspoon ground black pepper

½ teaspoon dried oregano

½ teaspoon Sea salt

¼ teaspoon ground black pepper

Vegetables:

2 tablespoon organic coconut oil

1 yellow bell pepper, trimmed, deseeded and sliced

1 red bell pepper, trimmed, deseeded and sliced

1 yellow onion, trimmed, peeled and sliced into thin slices

1 garlic clove, minced

5 ounces shiitake mushrooms

2 green onions, green part, sliced

1 cup vegetable broth

1 jalapeno, seeded and sliced thinly {leave the seeds if you like it HOT}

¼ cup chopped cilantro

1 avocado, peeled, seeded and thinly sliced

INSTRUCTIONS

1.   Place steak, lime juice and spices in a large bowl and toss together until steak is evenly coated.

2.   Set aside.

3.   Place a large, heavy skillet over medium-high heat, I used cast-iron. Add coconut oil to the pan and when melted add steak.

4.   Try to lay steak out so that it is in a single layer on the pan.

5.   Let steak sear 3-4 minutes, flip and cook the other side of steak for an additional 3-4 minutes, you want the outside to be completely seared. Remove steak from pan and set aside on a plate.

6.   Add onions, peppers, garlic and mushrooms to pan, tossing to coat. There should be enough juice from the steak to toss and coat your veggies. If not, add about ¼ cup of your vegetable broth. Try to scrape any excess brown bits that are stuck to the bottom of the pan. Toss your veggies until they start to soften, about 5 minutes. Add green onion, jalapeño, vegetable broth, steak and any juices that collected on the plate.

7.   Toss and cook for an additional 5-8 minutes.

8.   Remove from heat, toss cilantro on top as well as sliced avocado and additional jalapeño slices if you like.

9.   Serve with rice, fajitas or lettuce cups

11. SWEET POTATO AND PINEAPPLE BEEF BOWLS

A hearty salad bowl can be the perfect quick fix when you don't feel like getting out the pots and pans. This one gets its sweetness from pineapple and mango. Just be sure you opt for the real thing (not the canned versions) to avoid added sugars.

INGREDIENTS

For the Sweet Potato

3-4 large sweet potatoes, cut into 1-inch pieces

2 tablespoons olive oil

½ teaspoon salt

For the Pineapple Beef

1 tablespoon olive oil

1 pound lean ground beef (grass-fed if possible)

1 can 8oz crushed pineapple

1 teaspoon cumin

1 teaspoon garlic powder

1 teaspoon mild chili powder

½ teaspoon salt

For the Salsa

1 large mango, diced

2 avocados, diced

1 lime, juiced

¼ cup cilantro

¼ teaspoon salt

For the Bowls

5 oz baby spinach

Hot sauce (optional)

INSTRUCTIONS

1. Heat the oven to 400F.

2. Toss the sweet potatoes, 2 tablespoons olive oil, and ½ teaspoon salt together on a sheet pan.

3.   Roast for 15 minutes, flip the potatoes, then roast an additional 15 minutes or until golden brown and tender.

4.   Heat 1 tablespoon olive oil in a large saute pan. Add the beef, stirring to break into chunks. Sprinkle with cumin, garlic powder, mild chile powder, and ½ teaspoon salt. Cook 5-8 minutes or until the beef is browned and cooked through. Drain any extra fat, then add the pineapple and stir to combine. Turn the heat to low until ready to serve.

5.   Combine the mango, avocado, lime juice, cilantro, and salt in a large bowl. Stir to combine.

6.   Place the spinach, pineapple beef, and sweet potatoes in a bowl. Top with the mango, avocado salsa and hot sauce to taste.

12.   HEARTY VEGETABLE SOUP

With only one tablespoon of olive oil in the entire six-serving recipe, this may be a lower fat dish, but it's no "diet" soup. Packed with potatoes, lean ground beef, and chunky tomato sauce, it's a filling and nutritious dinner that's also easy to make in big batches.

INGREDIENTS:

1 Tablespoon olive oil

1 teaspoon minced garlic

1 to 1 1/2 pound lean ground beef or turkey

1/2 cup chopped onion

2 small potatoes or sweet potatoes, peeled and diced (can also substitute with cauliflower)

1 cup chopped celery

1 cup chopped carrots

1 (14.5 ounces) can rotel

1 (15 ounces) can tomato sauce

1 cup water

1 Tablespoon balsamic vinegar

1 - 2 teaspoons chili powder, more or less to taste

1/2 teaspoon kosher salt

1/2 teaspoon ground black pepper

3 tomatoes, diced (or substitute with 1-14 ounce can)

INSTRUCTIONS

1.	Heat the oil in a large pot over medium heat. Add the chopped onions and cook for 2 minutes. Stir in the garlic and cook for an additional 1 minute. Next, stir in the ground beef and cook until browned. Drain any remaining fat.

2.	Stir in potatoes, celery, and carrots, rotel, tomato sauce and water. Bring to a light simmer and then stir in the balsamic vinegar, chili powder, salt, pepper, and tomatoes.

3.	Reduce the heat to low and let simmer for about 30-45 minutes (or until the potatoes and carrots are forks tender), stirring occasionally.

4.	Top with fresh basil if desired.

## 13.	PORK ROAST WITH SWEET POTATOES, APPLES, AND ONION

Instead of sugary or preservative-laden applesauce, this Whole Diet makeover of the favorite pork and apple combo uses fresh chunks of the fruit, roasting it for a naturally sweet side to the protein. With diced sweet potato pitching in for some additional carb action, this meaty dish scores plenty of produce points.

INGREDIENTS

2 1/2 pound pork roast

2-4 apples, q uartered (used small gala, so used 4 apples, but if you use a larger apple like pink, lady or granny smith, I would only use 2)

2 sweet potatoes, cut into wedges

1 sweet onion, sliced

1/2 teaspoon sweet paprika

1/4 teaspoon cumin

1/4 teaspoon chili powder

Salt and pepper to taste

Olive oil (about 1/4 cup) enough to coat

INSTRUCTIONS

1. Preheat broiler to 500.

2. Rub pork with olive oil and season with salt and pepper.

3. Place on sheet tray and broil for 15 minutes, flipping halfway through cooking time (to get a nice color of meat).

4.   Meanwhile, chop apples, sweet potatoes, and onions. Toss in oil and spices.

5.   Arrange on sheet tray around the pork roast.

6.   Turn oven to down 450, and roast for 20-30 minutes, until apples and sweet potatoes are tender and meat reaches 120 degrees. This is a preference, most might say to cook for 140, but that is how you get dry pork. Allow the meat to rest at least 10 minutes before slicing and it will continue to cook and will be juicy! Return sliced pork and juices to the pan.

7.   Serve sliced pork with sweet potatoes, apples, onions and a simple salad.

14.   BALSAMIC AND BASIL MARINATED STEAK WITH ROASTED RED PEPPER PESTO

With just 10 main ingredients, skirt steak gets elevated from mere hunks of meat to seared strips loaded with flavor—and a ton of muscle-aiding iron. Soaked in a tangy marinade before generous dollops of the zippy (and nondairy!) red pepper pesto spoon on top.

INGREDIENTS

Steak Marinade

Balsamic basil marinated steak

1lb skirt steak (any steak)

1/4 cup balsamic vinegar

2 tbsp avocados or olive oil

1/4 cup fresh chopped basil (or 1 tbsp dried basil) 1 tbsp fresh minced garlic (or 1 tsp garlic powder

1 tsp pepper

1 tsp salt

1 tsp onion powder

Roasted Red Pepper Pesto

1/2 cup fresh basil, packed

1/2 cup roasted red peppers

1/4 cup pine nuts

1/4 cup olive oil

1 large garlic clove

1/2 tsp salt

1/2 tsp pepper

INSTRUCTIONS

1.   Marinate steak in a gallon sized plastic bag or Tupperware overnight or a minimum of 4 hours.

2.   Pan sear a steak in ghee or grill until cooked to your preference.

3.   While steak is cooking, prepare pesto.

4.   Add all pesto ingredients to food processor and pulse until combined into a pesto texture.

5.   Serve pesto on top of cooked steak.

15.   LAMB, MINT CHIMICHURRI, AND BUTTERNUT RICE

Cauliflower isn't the only veggie you can morph into rice-like granules! Butternut sq uash also makes an awesome substitute for the grain. Here it's made all buttery and wonderful with the addition of ghee (yup, enjoy ghee with glee!) and then topped with grilled lamb and drizzled with a fresh, herby chimichurri. This is dinner party-worthy stuff.

INGREDIENTS

2 pounds boneless lamb loin

Kosher salt

Freshly ground pepper

1 tbsp. olive oil

1 cup firmly packed fresh mint leaves

½ cup firmly packed flat-leaf parsley

2 garlic cloves, chopped

1 tsp. dried crushed red pepper

½ cup olive oil

⅓ cup red wine vinegar

1 butternut sq uash, peeled, seeded and roughly chopped (approximately 4 cups)

1 tablespoon ghee

3 cups beef broth

INSTRUCTIONS

1.   Make the chimichurri: put parsley, mint, garlic, red pepper flakes, olive oil and red wine vinegar in the bowl of a food processor and pulse 15-20 times until blended but not pureed. Pour into a bowl, cover and set aside.

2.   Prep the squash: Clean out the bowl of the food processor and add sq uash. Pulse 5-10 times until the sq uash resembles the size of rice. Set aside.

3.   Light charcoal grill or preheat a gas grill to 350-400 degrees. Add lamb loins and cover the grill. Grill for approximately 5 minutes on one side, then flip over and grill the other side approximately 3-5 minutes until the internal temp of the lamb reaches 130 degrees for medium rare.

4.   Remove loins from the grill, cover loosely with foil and let rest 5-7 minutes.

5.   While the lamb is resting, pour sq uash into a medium saucepan and add enough broth so the squash is just covered. Bring the sq uash mixture to a boil and add ghee. Reduce heat and simmer approximately 5-7 minutes until the sq uash is tender. Drain squash in a colander or strainer and place in a serving dish.

6.   Cut lamb against the grain into ¼" thick slices, then drizzle chimichurri on top. Serve immediately.

16.   TOMATO BASIL BEEF GOULASH WITH EGGPLANT

Trading in the dish's trademark paprika and caraway seeds for basil and garlic, and potatoes for eggplant. Whisking in the cream from the top of a can of coconut milk makes it extra luscious while keeping with the Whole Diet's no-dairy rule.

INGREDIENTS

2 tablespoons olive oil, divided

2 shallots, diced

4 garlic cloves, diced

1 lb ground beef

1 medium eggplant, cut into 1" cubes

1 (14oz) can diced tomatoes

⅓ cup fresh basil, diced

2 teaspoons salt

2 tablespoons tomato paste

¾ cup coconut cream (thick cream at the top of canned coconut milk)

INSTRUCTIONS

1.   Heat 1 tablespoon olive oil in a large saucepan over medium heat

2.   Add the shallots and garlic. Sauté for a few minute, until fragrant

3.   Add the ground beef and cook until brown

4.   In a separate saucepan, heat the other tablespoon of olive oil over medium heat and add the diced eggplant. Cook until soft, around 5 minutes

5.   Once the beef is browned, drain any excess grease, add the diced tomatoes (with juice), basil, and salt. Stir to combine, then add the coconut cream, tomato paste, and eggplant

6.   Serve immediately and garnish with more fresh basil

MEATLESS

17.   PALEO EGGS IN HELL

Eating clean, real foods on the Whole Diet doesn't mean splurging on pricey or obscure ingredients. Take this dinner, which turns a modest ingredient list into a protein-rich dish that, contrary to its name, tastes pretty heavenly.

INGREDIENTS

1 (28 oz) can diced tomatoes

1 tablespoon olive oil

1/2 white onion, diced

2 teaspoons red pepper flakes

1 tablespoon Italian seasoning

1/2 teaspoon salt

4 eggs

Parsley, for serving (optional)

INSTRUCTIONS

1. In a large cast iron skillet or Dutch oven, heat 1 tablespoon of olive oil over medium-high heat. Sauté the onion until soft, about 4 minutes. Stir in the red pepper flakes, salt, and Italian seasoning and stir until fragrant, about 1 minute.

2. Pour in the tomatoes and bring to a simmer for about 5 minutes. Make 4 divots in the sauce and crack an egg in each. Reduce the heat to low and cover. Cook for 3-5 minutes until the egg whites are set, but the yolk is still runny. Sprinkle with parsley and serve.

18. ZUCCHINI NOODLES WITH EVERYTHING PESTO AND FRIED EGGS

If spiralized zucchini never seemed like an adeq uate pasta alternative before, maybe this recipe will convince you. Lathered in a dairy-free pesto and topped with a fried egg, the noodles are every bit as tasty as real spaghetti, but with none of the gluten and a fraction of the carbs.

INGREDIENTS

For the everything pesto

1/4 Cup + 2 Tbsp Pine nuts toasted

1 Cup Lightly packed fresh herbs of choice, used basil

2 Scallions, trimmed and roughly chopped

1 clove Garlic, crushed

1/4 tsp Flaky sea salt or more to taste

3 Tbsp Extra-virgin olive oil

1 tsp Fresh lime or lemon juice

For the sq uash noodles and fried eggs

2 pounds of 3 zucchini, summer squash or cousa sq uash, julienned or spiralized (I used zucchini)

1/2 tsp Flaky sea salt or more to taste

3 tsp Ghee or extra-virgin olive oil

Freshly ground black pepper

2 Large eggs

INSTRUCTIONS

To make the everything pesto:

1.   Pulse 1/4 cup of the pine nuts, the herbs, scallion, garlic and salt in a food processor until coarsely chopped. Add the olive oil and lime juice and pulse again, scraping down the sides of the bowl as needed. Taste the pesto and add more salt if desired.

To make the sq uash noodles and fried eggs:

1.   Put the sq uash in a colander lined with paper towels. Toss with 1/2 tsp of salt and set aside for a few minutes, so the salt can draw some of the moisture out of the squash

2.   Heat 1 tsp of the ghee in a large skillet with a lid over medium-high heat. Add the squash noodles and cook, tossing frequently, until cooked to your liking. Take it off the heat and

add the pesto. Toss to combine, and season with salt and pepper to taste. Cover the skillet to keep the noodles, hot while you make the eggs.

3.   Heat the remaining 2 tsp of ghee in a medium-sized skillet over medium heat, and fry the eggs until cooked to your liking.

4.   Divide the noodles between 2 plates. Top each pile of noodles with a fried egg and 1 Tablespoon of pine nuts. Serve immediately.

19.   SLOW COOKER RATATOUILLE SOUP

With a whopping eight different veggies, this may as well be called "the one-stop stew for your daily recommended fiber and vitamin intake" (although "ratatouille soup" sounds much more appetizing). The produce is cooked down in a mix of its own juices and fruity olive oil, yielding a large batch that will have dinner covered for days.

INGREDIENTS

8 tomatoes, boiled, skinned and chopped

2 red bell peppers (chopped)

2 yellow bell peppers (chopped)

2 green bell peppers (chopped)

2 small zucchini (chopped)

1 yellow sq uash (chopped)

1 eggplant (peeled and cubed)

1 yellow onion (chopped)

1/4 cup olive oil

2 tsp minced garlic

2 T fresh basil, chopped

2 T fresh parsley

Sea salt to taste

INSTRUCTIONS

Throw everything in a slow cooker and cook for at least 6 hours. Cook on high for the first hour and then turn down to low for the remaining hours. Feel free to cook it longer than 6 hours if you like. I think the longer a soup cook, the more the flavors develop.

Notes: To peel the tomatoes, core them and place them in a saucepan of boiling water. After a minute or two, pull them out and place them in an ice water bath. The skin should easily come off. You can try leaving the skins on for this soup, but they may get tough while cooking so long. Don't throw the skins away, though. You can save them with all your other scraps for homemade vegetable broth. Enjoy!

20.   SWEET POTATO AND KALE GRATIN

This gratin may be grain-free, gluten-free, and dairy-free, but it makes no compromises when it comes to flavor. A coconut milk-based cream sauce, fragrant with nutmeg, and an entire head of garlic. Gets slathered generously between layers of sweet potato disks and kale for a one-pan dinner that's light and decadent all at once.

INSTRUCTIONS

For the roasted garlic

1 head garlic

1/2 teaspoon olive oil

For the gratin:

4 tablespoons ghee (melted) or olive oil, divided

1 bunch kale, tough stems removed, chopped

3 pounds sweet potatoes, peeled and thinly sliced into 1/8″ thick rounds

1/4 cup chicken or vegetable stock

1 and 1/2 cups coconut milk (one 14.5 ounce can)

1 teaspoon salt, or to taste

Freshly ground black pepper, to taste

1/4 teaspoon freshly grated nutmeg

INSTRUCTIONS

1.   Preheat the oven to 400. Cut the top off the head of garlic so the tops of all the cloves are exposed, and drizzle the cut side with the olive oil. Wrap the head in tinfoil and place it right on your oven rack. Roast for about 45 minutes, or until the cloves are very soft when squeezed or pierced with a fork. Let cool for a few minutes, then squeeze each clove out of its peel and set aside in a medium bowl.

2.   Meanwhile, steam the kale until wilted, 2-3 minutes. You can use a metal strainer set over a saucepan of similar size

if you don't have a steamer. Put an inch or two of water in the saucepan, bring it to a boil, set the strainer with the kale on top, and cover. When the kale is wilted, set it aside to cool.

3.   Leave the oven at 400, and grease the bottom and sides of a 9×13″ glass baking dish with two tablespoons of the ghee or olive oil.

4.   Layer half the sweet potato slices in the bottom of the baking dish in overlapping rows. Squeeze the excess water from the kale and sprinkle it evenly on top of the sweet potatoes. Top with a little salt & pepper. Layer the remaining sweet potato slices on top of the kale.

5.   Add the coconut milk, stock, salt, pepper, and nutmeg to the bowl with the roasted garlic. Process with an immersion blender (or transfer to your regular blender to puree) until smooth. Pour the sauce evenly over the potatoes, and drizzle the remaining two tablespoons of ghee or oil on top.

6.   Cover the dish with tinfoil and bake for 25 minutes, then remove the tinfoil and bake for another 20-25 minutes, or until the sweet potatoes are tender. If you'd like to brown the top of your gratin a little more, set the oven to broil and place the gratin under the broiler for 1-2 minutes (don't walk away!). Let the gratin sit for 10 minutes before slicing and serving.

Conclusion

Always remember that the purpose of day by day diet programs is to help you burn more body fats while decreasing your intake of calories.

So, to help your fat burning diet program, focus on eating foods that will make you feel full without eating in large q uantities. Bread and pastas made out of whole grains are excellent examples of this. Fortunately, whole grain products can be purchased at any supermarket.

But aside from whole grain products, you can also include other foods such as nuts, artichokes, lettuce, chicken meat, etc., which are also proven to be effective in helping you lose weight.

When undergoing a day by day diet program, always check your motivation for losing body fat. Because, in the end, no one can actually force you to lose weight and stick to your fat burning diet program but yourself.

50836558R00062

Made in the USA
San Bernardino, CA
05 July 2017